# The Sun Salutation Exercise

## (Surya Namaskara)

*Burton Milward, Jr.*

**Line Drawings by Dudley Zopp**

AuthorHouse™
1663 Liberty Drive
Bloomington, IN 47403
www.authorhouse.com
Phone: 1-800-839-8640

First published by AuthorHouse 4/28/2009

ISBN: 978-1-4389-4764-8 (sc)

Printed in the United States of America
Bloomington, Indiana

This book is printed on acid-free paper.

Additional copies of this book are available from authorhouse.com.

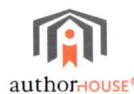

authorHOUSE®

# Contents

# Introduction

*Surya Namaskara* means Sun Salute or Sun Salutation. The term refers to a simple sequence of postures. This book is intended to lead the newcomer very gently into the practice of *Surya Namaskara*.

# Simple and Easy

One simple sequence of twelve postures provides more benefits more easily than any other exercise ever developed in human history.

Ask experienced Yoga teachers about the Sun Salute exercise, *Surya Namaskara*. They will praise *Surya Namaskara* for its many, many benefits, gained easily and quickly. The Sun Salute exercise is for young and old alike — men, women, and children.

The sequence consists of seven different stretching postures, five of which are then repeated in reverse order, for a total of twelve postures in all.

# Origin

In the dawn of history, a saint stood naked on the banks of the sacred Ganges, facing east as the sun rose over vast Himalayan mountains. Palms together, he stood at peace, filled only with reverence for *Surya's* light and warmth — life itself. He breathed morning air rich in *prana* (vitality). He began in the most natural way the stretching sequence described in this book.

# Vision

*Surya Namaskara* realigns us with the source of light, the sun, the pure light within us.

Performing *Surya Namaskara*, we enliven our experience of the life energy, the same experience of saints performing these postures again and again at the foothills of the Himalayas.

Although not exactly at the foothills of the Himalayas, yet facing the same morning sun, we partake of the same timeless cycle, celebrate the source of life, nourish, purify, and connect. We prepare to salute the sun.

Barefoot or in our favorite socks, on a grass lawn, on a sandy beach or a soft carpet, our palms joined in front of our chests, we stand beside each other in a respectful, peaceful posture. Sharing that moment of pleasant immersion in silence, we enjoy the warm light that unites. Eyes closed, our spines straight, in a relaxed pose of balance and stability, we absorb this state of tranquility amplified by each other's presence.

As we stretch upward, our clasped palms separate and open to the sun. We inhale the fresh morning air, looking into the unbounded sky. Our bodies arch back as a gentle breeze caresses our extended torsos. The vital energy enlivens our spine and chest.

We perform the postures of the Sun Salute exercise in sequence, one pose flowing into the next. The postures connect the sun and earth and soul, convey a feeling of wholeness greater than our individual selves. We gaze into the distance. We enjoy stretching into that greater wholeness.

*Surya* illuminates our faces. We surrender into the postures. We honor the sun. We pay homage to the life giving and life sustaining light of the universe. Finally, our bodies stand straight again in reverence to *Surya*, as our palms unite level with our chests representing the union of the inner and outer light.

As we perform the Sun Salute exercise together, the harmony of the sequence and the unity of the motion create a feeling of deeper connection between us.

Performing *Surya Namaskara* in unison removes tension and rigidity on the level of the body. As the mind and body connect, the mind becomes more relaxed and fluid. Such a mind opens itself easily to the experience of union with universal divine aspects of nature.

When we perform *Surya Namaskara* in unison, a deeper level of unity is experienced between us. The liveliness of subtle energy that is created becomes more palpable. The benefits multiply. As we rest at the end, easily lying on our backs beside each other, our connectedness with universal divine aspects of nature, and therefore our mutual connectedness, stabilizes on an ever-higher level.

This essential reverence for *Surya* as the divine light of life translates itself spontaneously into reverence for each other, as our individual love transforms itself into divine love.

Saluting the sun, we salute the divine soul within each other.

# Now for You

Into this timeless tradition, now you are born. Take this experience, benefit from it. This gift passes through others to you.

# Regular Practice

Regular practice of the Sun Salute postures results in excellent body tone, massaged inner organs and muscle groups, and a lively, vital central nervous system.

# Surya Namaskara

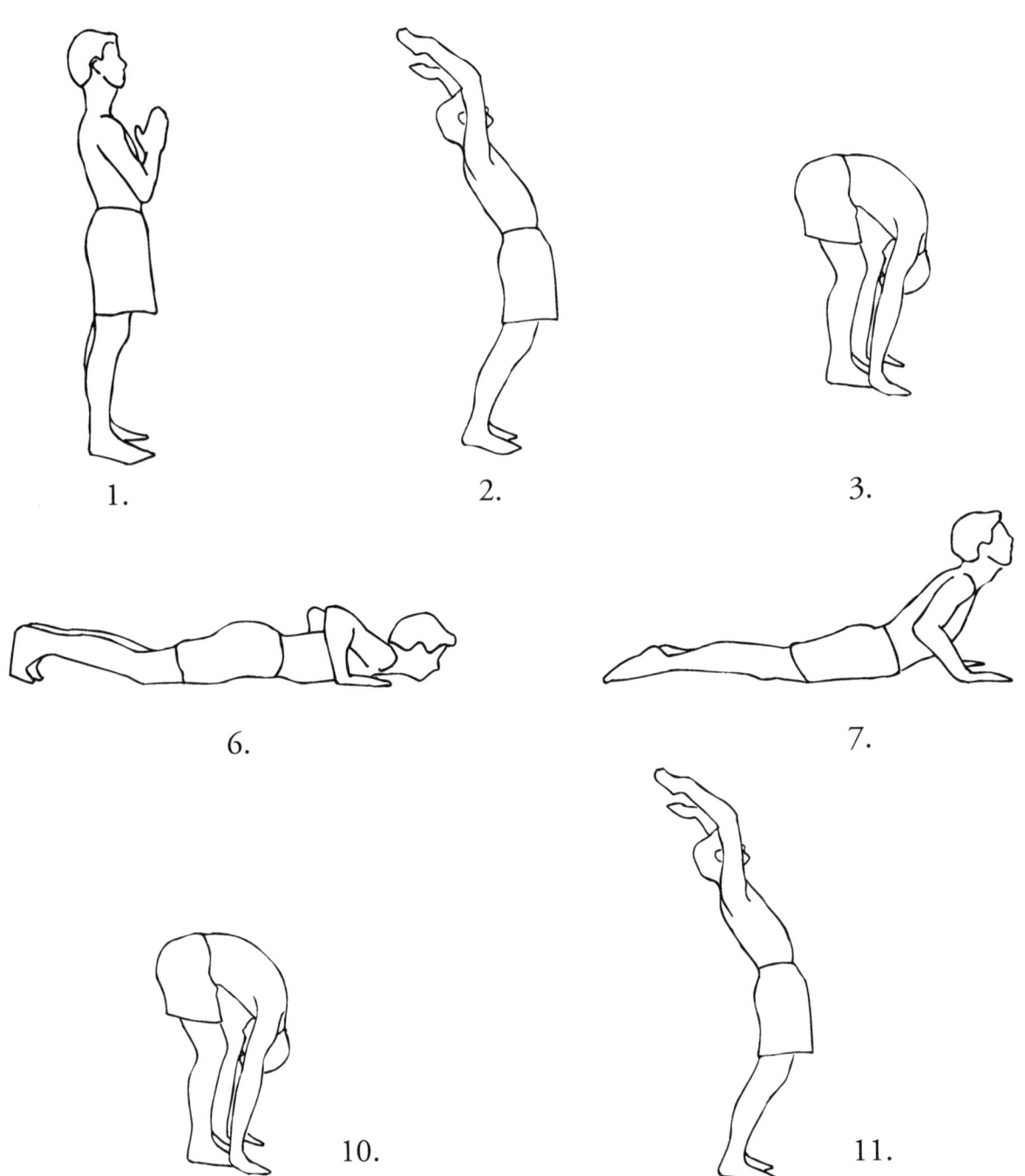

1.

2.

3.

6.

7.

10.

11.

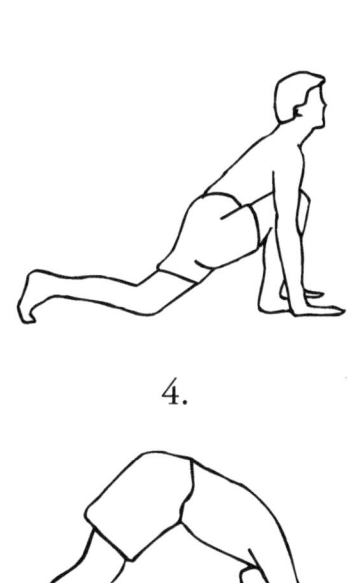

4.

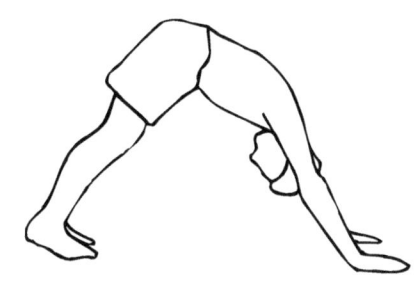

5.

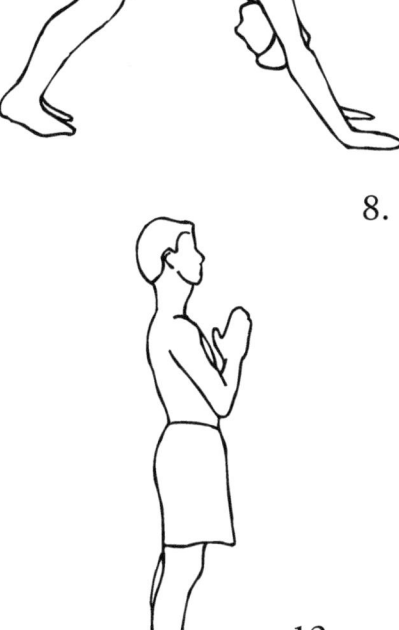

8.

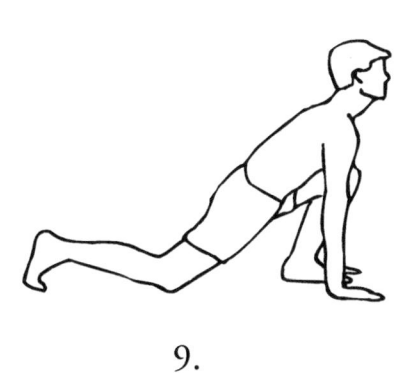

9.

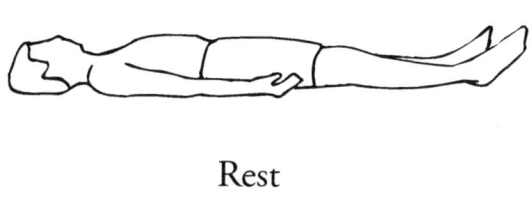

12.

Rest

11

# 1. Tradition

Although not considered part of traditional Hatha Yoga,[1] the Sun Salute exercise has been practiced since time immemorial by saints and devotees in India. The Sun Salute exercise expresses reverence to the sun as the provider of light and warmth, on whose presence all life on earth depends.

Today, the twelve successive positions of the Sun Salute exercise prepare the mind and body for life in our modern context:

> Modern life is exceedingly wearing; the noise, the excitement, the hurry, the competition, irregular hours, hard study, anxieties, worry, lack of proper food and exercise make a heavy tax on the constitution soon resulting in a breakdown of health. One can, however, be unaffected by these evils of modern civilization, if one should perform the *Surya Namaskara* exercise daily and take care of the diet, and make proper use of sunshine and open air.[2]

The simple rhythm of the Sun Salute exercise is available to women, men, children, young and old alike. It is the best and most economical tool for health widely available. It is designed to help everyone cope with the inevitable rigors of modern life.

The Rig Veda, ancient scripture, declares that "Surya is the Soul, both of the moving and unmoving beings."[3] The sun is revered as a symbol of health and immortality.[4]

---

1       Samskrti and Judith Franks, *Hatha Yoga: Manual Two*, Himalayan International Institute (Honesdale, Pennsylvania 1978), p. 28; Samskrti and Veda, *Hatha Yoga: Manual I*, Himalayan International Institute of Yoga Science and Philosophy (Honesdale, Pennsylvania 1979), p. 42; Swami Satyananda Saraswati, *Asana, Pranayama, Mudra, Bandha*, Bihar School of Yoga (Monghyr, Bihar, India 1973), p. 107.

2       Yogiraj Sri Swami Satchidananda, *Integral Hatha Yoga*, Holt, Rinehart and Winston (New York 1974), p. 25, quoting the King of Aundh, India (1940).

3       Lucy Lidell, *The Sivananda Companion to YOGA*, Simon and Schuster (New York 1983), p. 34.

4       *Id.*

# 2. Guidelines

An ideal morning routine begins with *Surya Namaskara*.

*Surya Namaskara* loosens up the whole body. It removes sleepiness. It stretches the spine and limbs.

Wear light clothing for *Surya Namaskara*. Practice on a clean, level surface, indoors or outdoors. Spread out a towel or blanket if desired. If practicing indoors, be sure to open a window for fresh air.

Start slowly, avoiding strain. Listen to your body as you begin to practice the sequence of twelve positions, each flowing into the next in one graceful, continuous movement. During the first week, become familiar with the positions only — the twelve postures and the sequence of the postures. After that, you can coordinate your breathing with the postures.

At the beginning, the twelve postures may seem separate to you, but soon these positions will blend into one continuous movement. You'll enjoy observing how each posture counterbalances the one before, stretching your body in a different way, alternately expanding and contracting the chest to regulate breath.

Don't strive for instant perfection. *Surya Namaskara* nurtures our growth with its constant potential for improvement. The more you practice *Surya Namaskara*, the more you'll enjoy it. The positions are never forced, never performed in a competitive way. Everyone performs within their own physical capabilities.

Each position should be held for three to five seconds. Begin by trying three seconds for each posture throughout the sequence.

Each "sequence" has twelve positions. Two sequences make one "set." Begin with two or three sets each morning, thereafter increasing the number according to your comfort and enjoyment. Many Yoga teachers recommend twelve sets daily. Others recommend a wide range of from two "sequences" to an extreme of three-hundred "sequences" daily.[5]

After you have performed several complete sets, lie down on your back, arms at your sides with palms facing up, allowing your body to relax. Close your eyes and rest for two minutes or more, breathing easily. This is very important, to fully relax lying down, so that the benefits of *Surya Namaskara* settle into your physiology.

Now you are ready to perform action, be it Yoga postures, or work or play.

---

5    James Hewitt, *The Complete Yoga Book*, Cresset Press (London 1990), p. 263.

# Three Points of Caution

1. If at any time you begin breathing or perspiring heavily or feel fatigued, stop the practice. Lie down and rest for a few minutes until your breathing returns to normal. Then resume the practice easily, without forcing, or begin again tomorrow. The guideline is comfortable practice.

2. If you are suffering from a bad back or knee injuries, or any medical condition such as high blood pressure or heart trouble, postpone the practice of *Surya Namaskara,* and be sure to consult your physician.

3. Some instructors recommend that women postpone the practice of the Sun Salute exercise entirely during the menstrual cycle and pregnancy. Other instructors recommend postponing the practice after the fourth month of pregnancy. Use your own best judgment, and be sure to consult your physician.

# 3. Names of the Twelve Positions

1. Pranamasana (salutation position)
2. Hasta Uttanasana (raised-arms position)
3. Padahastasana (hand-to-foot position)
4. Ashwa Sanchalanasana (equestrian position)
5. Parvatasana (mountain position)
6. Ashtanga Namaskara (eight-limbs position)
7. Bhujangasana (cobra position)
8. Parvatasana (mountain position)
9. Ashwa Sanchalanasana (equestrian position)
10. Padahastasana (hand-to-foot position)
11. Hasta Uttanasana (raised-arms position)
12. Pranamasana (salutation position)

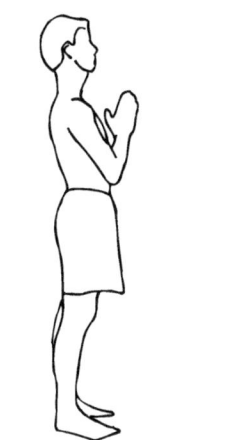
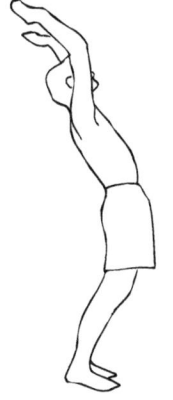
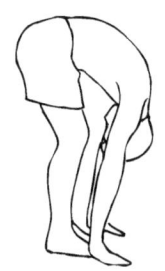
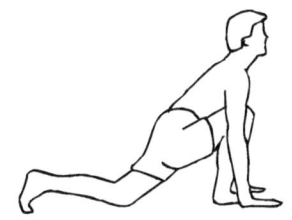

1. Pranamasana.  2. Hasta Uttanasana  3. Padahastasana  4. Ashwa Sanchalanasana

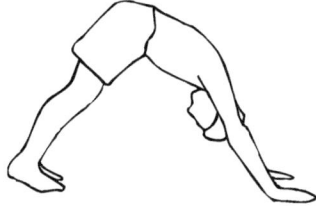
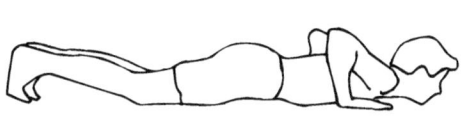
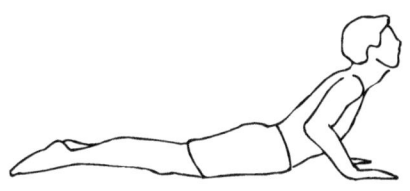

5. Parvatasana  6. Ashtanga Namaskara  7. Bhujangasana

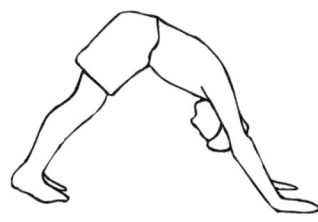
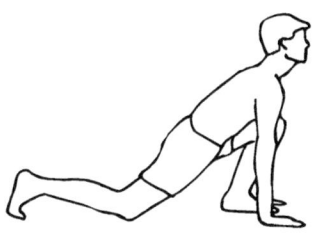
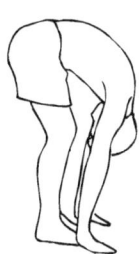

8. Parvatasana  9. Ashwa Sanchalanasana  10. Padahastasana

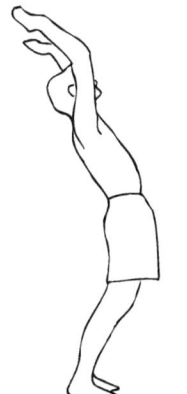
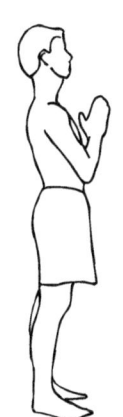
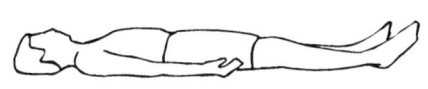

11. Hasta Uttanasana  12. Pranamasana  Shavasana

# 4. The Twelve Positions Described

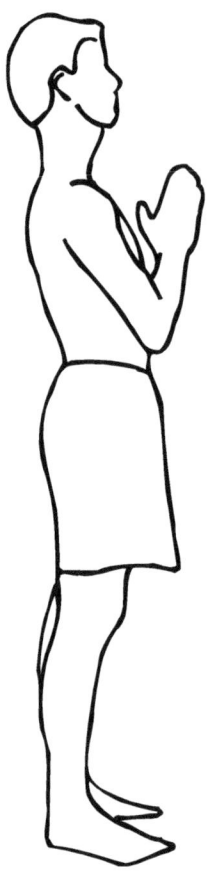

# 1. Pranamasana (salutation position)

Stand erect with feet together. Place palms together in front of chest, fingers pointing upward. Relax the whole body.

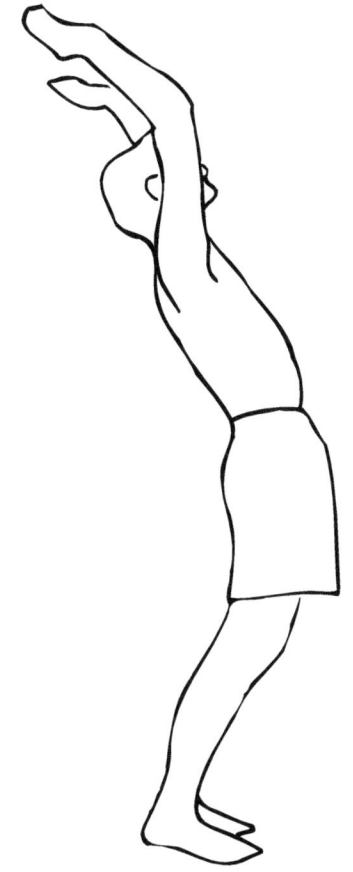

# 2. Hasta Uttanasana (raised-arms position)

Raise both arms high above the head and stretch the arms up and backward. Extend the arms fully. Arch the head and upper body backward from the waist. Arch the spine and bend backward without straining. As you reach up and arch back, the chest expands and you breathe in naturally.

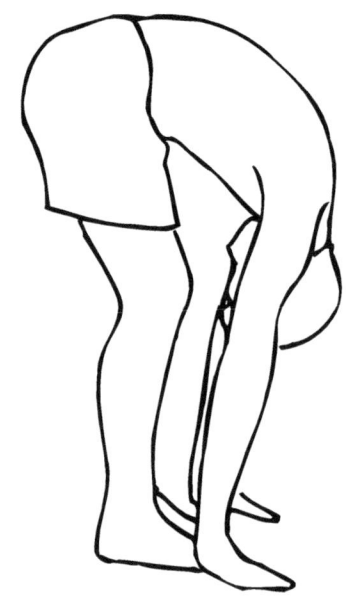

# 3. Padahastasana (hand-to-foot position)

Bend down from the waist until hands and fingers touch the ground. Ideally, the palms are flat on the ground with fingers pointing forward beside the feet. Be sure to *allow the knees to bend freely* as necessary. Try to touch the forehead to the legs as nearly as possible, but without straining. With regular practice, the legs and spine will naturally experience increased flexibility.

If you cannot place your palms on the ground without bending your legs at the knees, then *bend your legs at the knees*. The palms will remain unmoved, in this same place on the ground, as the limbs and body stretch through the next seven positions, almost the entire sequence!

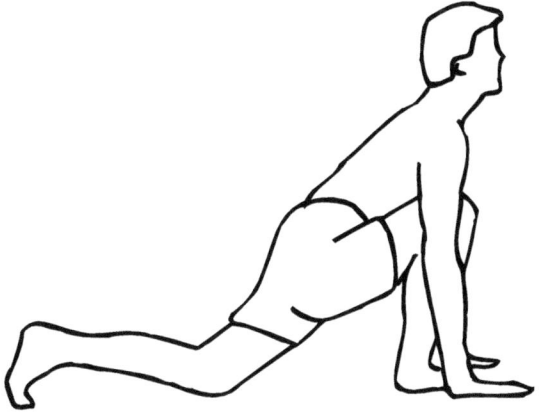

# 4. Ashwa Sanchalanasana (equestrian position)

Stretch the left leg back as far as possible, with the left knee touching the ground. The hip joint and muscles should be stretched as fully as comfortable.

Bend the right leg at the knee, without moving the right foot from its place in the previous position. The arms remain straight, leaving the hands in the same place as in the previous position. Arch the chest forward and up, extending the spine as completely as comfortable. Look up, way up.

The essence of this equestrian position is the extension of the spine. Maximize this extension, and enjoy the way it feels.

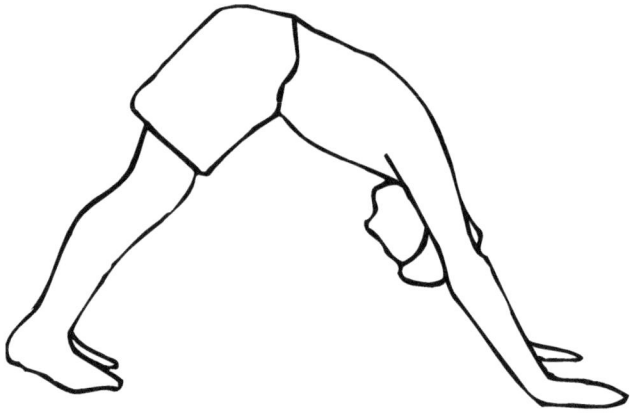

# 5. Parvatasana (mountain position)

Straighten the right leg and bring the right foot back beside the left foot. Raise the hips and buttocks as high as possible, lowering the head between the straightened arms, so that the body forms a triangle with the ground. The hands remain in the same place as in the previous position.

Your whole body stretches. Keep your heels in contact with the ground as much as is comfortable. Enjoy the gentle tautness of your leg muscles, especially your calves.

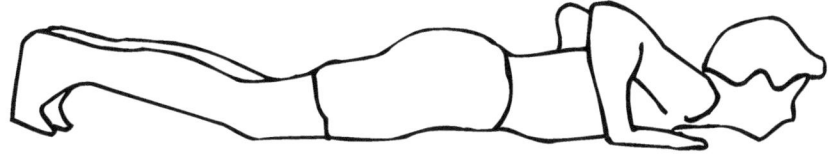

# 6. Ashtanga Namaskara (eight-limb position)

Lower the knees, then the chest, then the chin to the ground, so that only the toes, the knees, the chest, chin and hands touch the ground. The hands remain unmoved from the previous position. The hips and stomach should be slightly above the ground. The elbows and arms are bent and close to the body.

This position is called the *ashtanga*, or eightfold, salutation because eight parts of your body touch the ground: toes, knees, palms, chest, and chin.

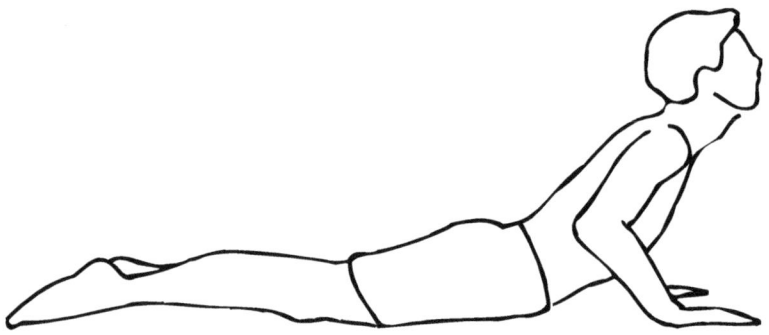

# 7. Bhujangasana (cobra position)

Lower hips and stomach to the ground. Stretch the chest, shoulders, neck, and head upwards, arching the upper body backward from the waist. The legs and feet are extended together and relaxed on the ground. Straighten the arms, balancing the upper body as it arches backward. Palms remain unmoved on the ground. The elbows remain slightly bent beside the body. The strength of the back, not the arms, arches the upper torso up and backward.

This is not a head-and-neck exercise. This is not a pushup. This is an arching-of-the-back position. Let your back muscles and spine arch your body and head upward from the waist. Use the muscles of your back. Use your arms and hands only for balance.

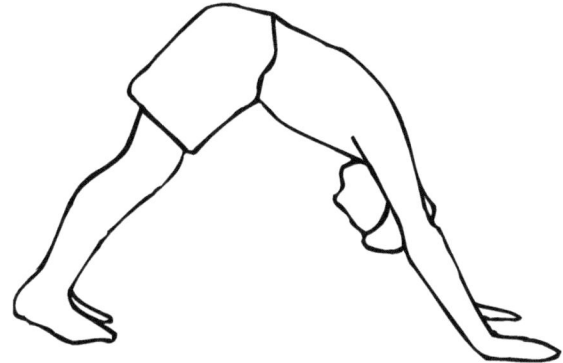

# 8. Parvatasana (mountain position)

Without moving the palms from their place on the ground, raise the hips and buttocks as high as possible, lowering the head between the straightened arms, so that the body forms a triangle with the ground. This is the same posture as Position 5.

Your whole body stretches. Keep your heels in contact with the ground as much as is comfortable. Enjoy again the tautness of your leg muscles.

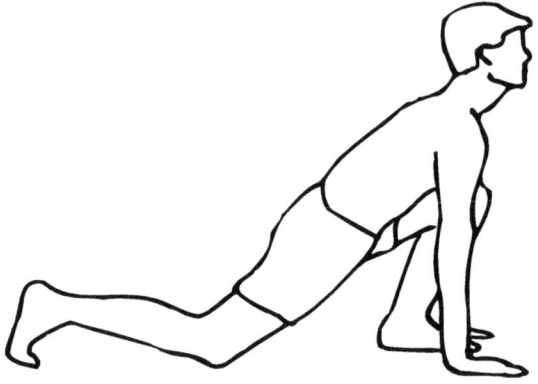

# 9. Ashwa Sanchalanasana (equestrian position)

This posture is the same as Position 4, except that the position of the legs is reversed, to ensure a balanced exercise.

Stretch the right leg back as far as possible, with the right knee touching the ground. The hip joint and muscles should be stretched as fully as comfortable. Bend the left leg at the knee and bring the left foot forward between the hands. The arms remain straight, leaving the palms flat on the ground, unmoved.

Arch the chest forward and up, extending the spine as completely as comfortable. Look up, way up. The essence of this equestrian position is the extension of the spine. Extend your spine, arching your chest forward and up. Enjoy the way it feels.

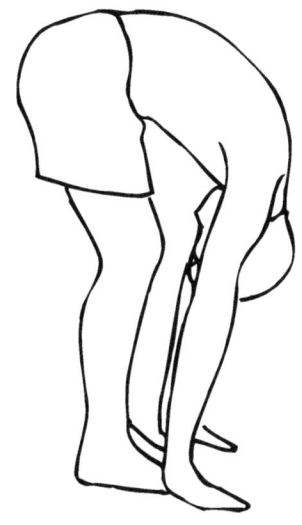

# 10. Padahastasana (hand-to-foot position)

Bring the right foot forward beside the left foot as the hands and fingers continue to touch the ground, with legs straightened. Ideally, the palms are flat on the ground. Be sure to *allow the knees to bend freely* as necessary. Try to touch the forehead to the legs as nearly as possible, but without straining. This posture is the same as Position 3.

If you cannot place your palms on the ground without bending your legs at the knees, then *bend your legs at the knees.*

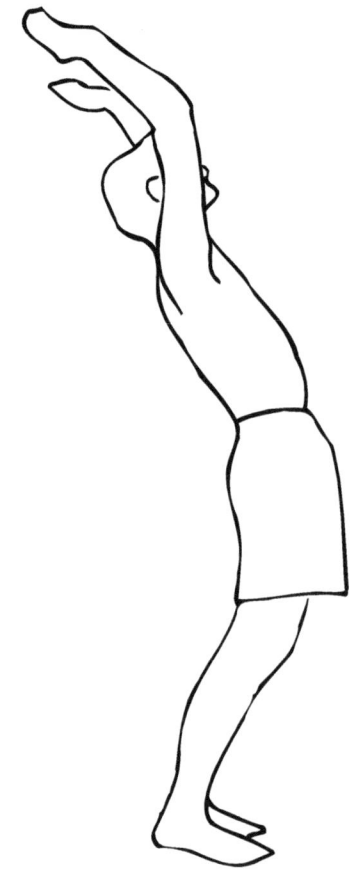

# 11. Hasta Uttanasana (raised-arms position)

Stand erect. Raise both arms high above the head and stretch the arms up and backward. Extend the arms fully. Arch the head and upper body backward from the waist. Arch the spine and bend backward without straining.

As you reach up and lean back, the chest expands and you breathe in naturally.

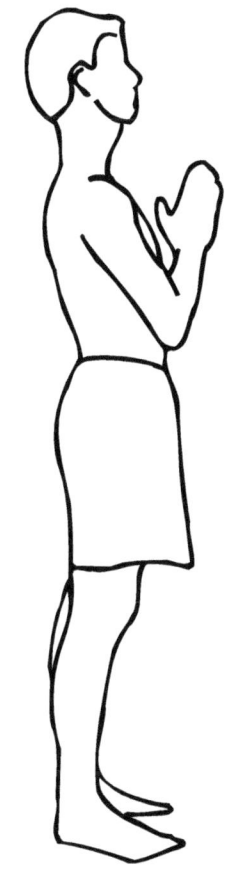

# 12. Pranamasana
# (salutation position)

Standing erect, with feet together, lower your hands and allow the palms to come together in front of your chest, fingers pointing upward. This is the final posture. It is the same as Position 1. This same standing salutation posture becomes the first position for the next sequence.

Remember to relax your whole body.

# Shavasana (corpse position)

After you have completed as many Sun Salutation "sets" as are comfortable for you, be sure to lie down on your back, eyes closed, with arms at your sides and palms facing up, for two or three minutes, breathing naturally and easily. Now relax. This corpse posture, or *shavasana*, allows your body and mind to completely integrate the benefits of *Surya Namaskara*.

# 5. Breathing

After you learn the positions and their sequence, then you can synchronize your breathing with the postures of the Sun Salute exercise.

1. Salutation ................................................. Normal, relaxed breathing
2. Raised Arms ............................................. Inhale
3. Hand to Foot ........................................... Exhale
4. Equestrian .............................................. Inhale
5. Mountain ................................................ Exhale
6. Eight Limbs ............................................. No breathing (glide quickly into next position)
7. Cobra .................................................... Inhale
8. Mountain ................................................ Exhale
9. Equestrian .............................................. Inhale
10. Hand to Foot .......................................... Exhale
11. Raised Arms ........................................... Inhale
12. Salutation ............................................. Normal, relaxed breathing

Be sure to either inhale or exhale, as appropriate, with each position. That is, don't breathe in and out within the same position.

One of the foremost exponents of the proper practice of *Surya Namaskara* describes its breathing experience as follows. "Inhale to extend your spine vertically or to open, lengthen, or fully elongate the body. Exhale to bend or fold the body, creating a flexing of the spine."[6]

Please refer to the figure drawings marked with breathing guidelines on the next page.

---

6    Deepak Chopra, M.D., *Perfect Health: The Complete Mind/Body Guide*, Harmony Books (New York 1990), p. 269.

# Breathing

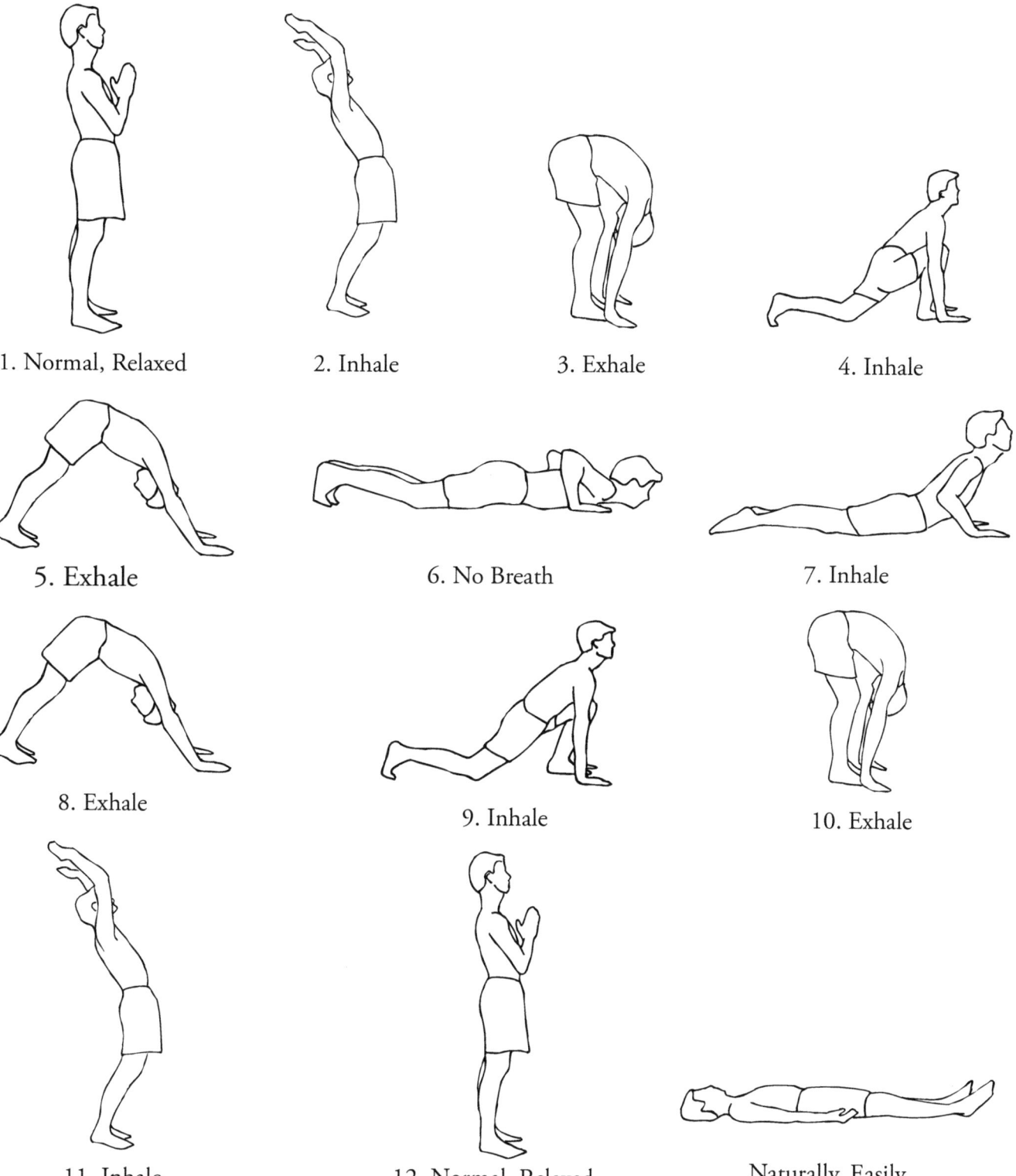

1. Normal, Relaxed

2. Inhale

3. Exhale

4. Inhale

5. Exhale

6. No Breath

7. Inhale

8. Exhale

9. Inhale

10. Exhale

11. Inhale

12. Normal, Relaxed

Naturally, Easily

# 6. Benefits

*Surya Namaskara* has been described as "a very complete combination of bodily postures and breathing."[7] It gives "a yoga session in miniature."[8] It "has a very warming effect on the entire body far superior to any athletic limbering up."[9]

Practiced in the morning, *Surya Namaskara* provides a graceful and thorough transition from the inactive state of sleep to the active state of waking.

*Surya Namaskara* simultaneously integrates the whole physiology of mind, body, and breath. It combines bodily postures and breathing with a reverential attitude of mind.

*Surya Namaskara* strengthens and stretches all the major muscle groups. It tones arm and leg muscles and lubricates the joints. It conditions the spine to be supple and healthy. It massages the internal organs by alternately stretching and compressing the abdomen. Regular practice tones the digestive organs and improves the elimination process.

*Surya Namaskara* makes the heart and lungs stronger by increasing blood flow and circulation throughout the body. It synchronizes the breath with physical movements to ensure, at least for a few minutes daily, that practitioners breathe as they should — deeply and rhythmically. "Each position counteracts the one before, stretching the body in a different way and alternately expanding and contracting the chest to regulate the breathing."[10] This deep and rhythmic breathing removes stagnant air from the lungs and replaces it with fresh, oxygen-rich air. The influx of fresh, oxygen-rich blood to the brain increases clarity of mind.

7    Yogiraj Sri Swami Satchidananda, *Integral Hatha Yoga*, Holt, Rinehart and Winston (New York 1974), p. 25.
8    William Zorn, *Body Harmony: The Easy Yoga Exercise Way*, Hawthorn Books (New York 1971), p. 7.
9    Kevin and Venika Kingsland, *Complete Hatha Yoga*, Arco Publishing (New York 1983), p. 81.
10   Lucy Lidell, *The Sivananda Companion to YOGA*, Simon and Schuster (New York 1983), p. 34.

*Surya Namaskara* naturally and easily removes psychosomatic tensions. The sequence of postures gently stimulates nerve connections throughout the whole body, allowing them to relax, or function more harmoniously, and become revitalized. *Surya Namaskara* "has a very powerful influence on all the systems of the body: endocrinal, circulatory, respiratory, digestive, etc., and helps to bring them into balance with each other. Many diseases are caused when one or more of these systems are out of balance with each other; *Surya Namaskara*, by putting them in equilibrium, helps to remedy many ailments."[11]

It is claimed that *Surya Namaskara* is "a hymn of happiness"[12] which "will help you maintain your vitality and keep your youthful looks till a ripe old age."[13]

11      Swami Satyananda Saraswati, *Asana, Pranayama, Mudra, Bandha*, Bihar School of Yoga (Monghyr, Bihar, India 1973), p. 121.

12      Andre Van Lysebeth, *YOGA Self-Taught*, Harper & Row (New York 1971), p. 232.

13      William Zorn, *Body Harmony: The Easy Yoga Exercise Way*, Hawthorn Books (New York 1971), p. 8.

# 7. Reverential Thoughts

When the positions of the Sun Salute exercise have been learned, when the sequence of the positions flows effortlessly, when the postures are synchronized with the breathing, then the deeper, inward stroke of reverential thoughts may be introduced.

With reverential thoughts for the sun, for the life the sun gives, for the pure light within, *Surya Namaskara* is transformed from an ordinary muscular exercise into a whole experience embracing devotional as well as physical realities.

One commentator sets forth a traditional sequence of thoughts parallel to the sequence of positions performed in the Sun Salute exercise.

> With hands in prayer I face the sun, feeling love and joy in my heart. I reach out and let the sun fill me with warmth. I bow before the sun's radiance and place my face to the ground in humble respect. I lift my face to the sun and then remember, to achieve such heights, I must be as the dust of the earth. I stretch up towards its light trying to reach the greatest heights and again surrender. I stand tall as I remember the true sun is within me.[14]

In the Valmiki *Ramayana*, the great rishi Vishwamitra revealed a beautiful sun prayer to Lord Rama:

> I always adore Surya, the sun, the beautiful lord of the world, the immortal quintessence of Vedanta, the auspicious, the absolute Brahmanic knowledge, the lord of the devas, the ever-pure, the one true consciousness of the world, the

---

14    Samskrti and Veda, *Hatha Yoga: Manual I*, Himalayan International Institute of Yoga Science and Philosophy (Honesdale, Pennsylvania 1979), pp. 44–45.

lord of Indra, of the gods, of men and of the worlds, the very heart of Brahma, Vishnu and Shiva, the giver of light.[15]

Other contemplations, mantras, and recitations appear in the literature, but it is the reverential attitude itself, rather than these formulas, which ensures a complete and fulfilling practice of *Surya Namaskara.*

---

15    Swami Shivananda Saraswati, *Surya Namaskar: A Technique in Solar Vitalization*, Bihar School of Yoga (Monghyr, Bihar, India 1973), pp. 3–4.

# 8. Variations

**Variation One.** If you are feeling restless, perform *Surya Namaskara* slowly. Slow performance is a tool which may quiet your restlessness.

**Variation Two.** If you are feeling listless or drowsy, perform *Surya Namaskara* rapidly. Rapid performance is a tool which may restore alertness.

**Variation Three.** Experienced practitioners sometimes perform *Surya Namaskara* very quickly. The twelve positions remain the same, but the pace is quite rapid. The sequence flows without ever stopping. Breathing is not emphasized. Each "sequence" of twelve positions is completed in less than thirty seconds. A series of thirty-six quick "sets" in rapid succession each morning enhances aerobic benefits.

**Variation Four.** A more strenuous variation of *Surya Namaskara* is called the Hero Series. The first posture is the traditional salutation position, except that the feet are not together but widespread. The positions vary in greater degrees of difficulty as the sequence unfolds. An excellent discussion of the Hero Series is set forth in Samskrti and Judith Franks' *Hatha Yoga: Manual Two*, at pages 28–39.

**Variation Five.** You may create your own variation of the Sun Salute exercise, consciously enjoying the sun and your own flexibility. If it satisfies you, continue with it. Only be careful not to overexert yourself.

# Conclusion

Now enjoy performing the Sun Salute exercise!

Go ahead, nurture youthful suppleness in your spine. Firm and tone your whole body!

Do this in reverence for life and your expression of life. And then, when you have mastered *Surya Namaskara*, introduce others to this graceful practice and share with them its benefits.

*Namaste*

Lightning Source UK Ltd.
Milton Keynes UK
UKHW051622031119
352762UK00002B/27/P